HEALTHY EATING COOKBOOK FEMALE

Nourishing Recipes for Women: A Female focused, dietary nutrition guide, Wellness, Her Health Kitchen, cuisine Nutritious and Balanced meals

Brandon Oliver

TABLE OF CONTENTS

INTRODUCTION

This book invites you on a culinary exploration aimed at nurturing your body, mind, and spirit. It is a tribute to women who seek a harmonious and healthful life, craving tasty recipes that enhance their well-being.

As women, our bodies undergo various transformations from puberty to pregnancy, menopause, and beyond. These changes demand a diet abundant in vital nutrients. The goal of this cookbook is to present you with a selection of recipes tailored to support your health and vitality through every phase.

Within these pages, you'll discover a diverse array of nourishing and flavorful dishes that celebrate fresh, whole foods. From lively salads and comforting soups to satisfying mains and guilt-free desserts, each recipe is designed with your health as a priority.

Whether you're aiming to increase your energy levels, promote hormonal balance, or simply indulge in meals that bring joy, the Healthy Female Cookbook is your ultimate resource for wholesome recipes that cater to your distinct needs as a woman.

Let's embark on this journey together, embracing a lifestyle that respects and nurtures our bodies and minds, one delectable meal at a time.

CHAPTER 1
HEALTHY EATING

Defining healthy eating involves striking a balance in your food choices to nurture both your body and mind, ensuring they remain strong, energized, and properly nourished. Cultivating healthy eating habits is a fundamental aspect of self-care.

Key Guidelines for Healthy Eating

1. Consistency in Meals: Aim for three main meals a day (breakfast, lunch, and dinner) supplemented with 2-3 nutritious snacks whenever hunger strikes or between meals.

2. Diverse Food Selection: Consume a variety of foods from all food groups daily, including grains, fruits, vegetables, proteins, dairy, and healthy fats, to fulfill your nutritional requirements.

3. Mindful Eating: Listen to your body's cues, eating when hungry and stopping when feeling comfortably full.

Benefits of Healthy Eating

• Sustained Energy Levels

• Equate Vitamin and Mineral Intake

• Enhanced Physical Performance

• Optimal Growth Potential (especially for those still growing)

• Prevention of Unhealthy Eating Patterns like skipping meals and subsequent overeating

Tips for Practicing Healthy Eating

1. Meal Planning: Avoid skipping meals by planning meals and snacks in advance to maintain steady energy levels and promote overall health.

2. Prioritize Breakfast: Kick starts your day with a balanced breakfast to fuel your body and sustain focus throughout the day.

3. Eating Out: Be prepared when dining away from home by either packing nutritious foods or knowing where to find healthy options.

4. Cooking Techniques: Experiment with healthier cooking methods such as grilling, stir-frying, microwaving, baking, or boiling instead of deep-frying.

5. Flavor Enhancement: Use herbs, spices, citrus juices, or healthy oils to add flavor to your meals while reducing reliance on added fats and sugars.

6. Trim Fat: Go for lean cuts of meat and remove visible fat to reduce saturated fat intake while retaining flavor and nutrients.

7. Hydration: Stay adequately hydrated by consuming water throughout the day to support bodily functions and maintain energy levels.

8. Varied Fat Sources: Incorporate diverse fat sources like olive oil or canola oil for heart-healthy benefits and unique flavors.

9. Plant-Based Proteins: Experiment with Meatless Monday to include plant-based protein sources like soy, beans, and wheat gluten in your diet.

10. Mindful Eating Practices: Slow down, savor each bite, and pay attention to hunger and fullness cues to promote better digestion and satisfaction.

11. Embrace Variety: Avoid restrictive dieting mentalities and instead focus on balanced, sustainable lifestyle changes for long-term health and happiness.

12. Seek Professional Guidance: Consult a registered dietitian for personalized nutrition advice and support in making informed dietary choices.

Remember, while nutrition plays a crucial role in overall well-being, it's just one aspect of leading a fulfilling life.

CHAPTER 2

BALANCING HORMONES THROUGH DIET

Hormonal imbalances can lead to various health issues ranging from infertility to diabetes. However, incorporating specific foods into your diet can aid in balancing your hormones and ensuring proper bodily functions. We'll delve into which foods to prioritize for optimal hormone health.

When considering our dietary choices, hormones might not immediately come to mind. Nevertheless, hormones play a pivotal role in numerous bodily functions. Acting as chemical messengers within the endocrine system, hormones contribute to growth, metabolism, digestion, fertility, stress response, mood regulation, and more. When hormonal levels fluctuate excessively, it can result in conditions such as diabetes, weight fluctuations, infertility, and other health concerns.

The Influence of Diet on Hormones

Our food choices directly impact hormone production and signaling pathways. Hormones thrive on nutrients like healthy fats found in olive oil, avocado, nuts, and seeds, alongside abundant fiber from fruits and vegetables, and quality proteins such as eggs, fish, and meat. Conversely, substances like pesticides, alcohol, and artificial sweeteners can disrupt hormonal balance.

Caloric intake also plays a crucial role. Especially for women, whose bodies are highly sensitive to scarcity, insufficient calorie intake can trigger a down regulation of sex hormone production. Whether due to famine, war, or a restrictive diet, the body responds similarly.

Detecting Hormonal Imbalance

For women in their reproductive years, menstrual cycles can offer insight into hormonal balance. Symptoms like infertility, PMS, heavy or painful periods, and migraines may indicate hormonal imbalances. Additionally, sudden changes in weight or energy levels could signal such imbalances. However, definitive diagnosis typically requires testing.

Understanding Hormonal Functions

The human body contains more than 200 hormones, including well-known ones like estrogen, testosterone, cortisol, insulin, leptin, ghrelin, and thyroid hormones. These substances play crucial roles in controlling metabolism, fertility, and mood.

Metabolic Hormones

Insulin regulates blood sugar levels by facilitating the transfer of glucose from the bloodstream to cells for energy. It also stores excess sugar as fat.

Leptin, produced by fat cells, controls appetite and signals satiety to the brain.

Ghrelin, often referred to as the hunger hormone, triggers feelings of hunger and stimulates appetite.

Thyroid hormones T3 and T4 regulate weight, energy levels, temperature, and various physiological processes.

Reproductive Hormones

Estrogen, the primary female sex hormone, governs puberty changes, menstrual cycles, pregnancy maintenance, cholesterol levels, and bone density.

Testosterone, the primary male sex hormone, influences puberty changes, libido, bone density, and muscle strength in both genders.

Stress and Mood Hormones

Cortisol, the stress hormone, elevates blood pressure and heart rate during stressful situations.

Adrenaline, the fight or flight hormone, increases heart rate in response to stress.

Melatonin, the sleep-inducing hormone, prepares the body for sleep.

Optimal Foods for Hormonal Balance

Cruciferous vegetables, particularly broccoli and broccoli sprouts, support efficient estrogen metabolism in the liver. Other cruciferous veggies like cauliflower, Brussels sprouts, kale, cabbage, and bok choy offer similar benefits. Roasting them with olive oil enhances the absorption of vitamins A, D, E, and K, further aiding in hormonal balance.

Salmon and Albacore Tuna: Fats and cholesterol serve as the fundamental building blocks of hormones, essential for the synthesis of sex hormones like estrogen and testosterone. Opting for fats rich in omega-3 fatty acids while limiting saturated fats and eliminating trans fats is key. Foods such as salmon, canned albacore tuna, walnuts, flaxseed, olive oil, avocados, and chia seeds are excellent sources of omega-3s. Salmon, in particular, not only aids in stabilizing hunger hormones but also boasts high levels of vitamin D, crucial for regulating female testosterone levels. The beneficial fats present in fish contribute to enhanced hormonal communication, facilitating improved mood and cognitive function through interaction with the brain.

Avocados: Abundant in beta-sitosterol, avocados play a role in positively impacting blood cholesterol levels and cortisol balance. Moreover, the plant sterols present in avocados have an impact on estrogen and progesterone, which are essential hormones governing ovulation and menstrual cycles. Recent studies have shown that the combination of fat and fiber in avocados promotes the release of hormones associated with satiety, including peptide YY (PYY), cholecystokinin (CCK), and glucagon-like peptide 1 (GLP-1). Incorporating half an avocado into meals can prolong feelings of fullness, offering a satiating effect.

Fruits and Vegetables (Preferably Organic): Opting for organic fruits and vegetables is crucial due to the adverse effects of pesticides on fertility. Pesticides can act as hormone disruptors, mimicking or interfering with natural hormone actions in the body. Glyphosate, a well-known endocrine disruptor, is commonly found in non-organic produce. By choosing organic options, exposure to glyphosate and other harmful chemicals is significantly reduced, promoting hormonal balance and overall health.

High-Fiber Carbohydrates: A diet rich in fiber, derived from fruits, vegetables, and whole grains, aids in the elimination of excess hormones from the body. Lignans, abundant in flaxseed, facilitate the binding and removal of active estrogens, further contributing to hormonal balance. Incorporating non-starchy vegetables into most meals, along with a portion of starchy vegetables or whole grains, supports hormone regulation. Root vegetables like carrots, sweet potatoes, and squashes, along with beans and whole grains, are beneficial additions to promote hormonal equilibrium.

Prebiotics and Probiotics: Supporting gut health is essential for hormonal balance, as the gut serves as a significant endocrine organ. Prebiotic foods such as raw garlic, oats, asparagus, dandelion, almonds, apples, bananas, Jerusalem artichokes, and chicory nourish beneficial gut bacteria. Additionally, incorporating probiotic-rich foods like kimchi and yogurt promotes a healthy gut microbiome, fostering optimal hormone production and regulation.

Foods to Limit for Hormonal Balance
Processed Foods, Fried Foods, Sugar, and Artificial Sweeteners: Consuming less processed foods, fried items, sugar, and artificial sweeteners helps prevent hormonal imbalances. Research suggests that artificial sweeteners may alter gut bacteria, affecting hunger and satiety hormones like leptin and ghrelin.

Alcohol: Limiting alcohol consumption is essential for hormone balance, as it interferes with various hormonal processes, including blood sugar control and estrogen metabolism. Excessive alcohol intake is associated with an increased risk of breast cancer and other cancers. Women are advised to restrict themselves to one alcoholic beverage per day, while men should keep their consumption to a maximum of two drinks daily.

Lifestyle Factors Impacting Hormonal Balance

In addition to dietary considerations, maintaining adequate sleep, managing stress levels, and engaging in regular exercise are vital for hormone balance. Sleep deprivation can lower testosterone levels in men and disrupt hunger-regulating hormones like leptin and ghrelin. Chronic stress leads to elevated cortisol levels, which can negatively affect digestion, immunity, and blood pressure. Prioritizing activities like exercise, meditation, and sufficient sleep can help manage stress levels and promote hormonal equilibrium. Additionally, certain foods such as chocolate can boost mood-regulating hormones like norepinephrine and serotonin, further supporting overall well-being.

Finally, hormones play a crucial role in various bodily functions, including growth, metabolism, fertility, stress response, mood regulation, and appetite control. A balanced diet comprising fruits, vegetables, whole grains, healthy fats, and protein is essential for maintaining hormonal equilibrium. Conversely, inadequate calorie intake, unhealthy fats, and lack of fiber can disrupt hormone balance, potentially leading to conditions such as obesity, diabetes, infertility, and cancer. Lifestyle factors including sleep, stress management, exercise, and dietary choices all contribute to overall hormonal health.

CHAPTER 3

IMPROVE YOUR REPRODUCTIVE HEALTH WITH FOOD

Struggling to conceive can be incredibly challenging, but it's a journey many couples face. In the United States, about one in eight couples encounter difficulties with conception or maintaining a pregnancy. Despite these obstacles, there are actionable steps both partners can take to enhance their chances of conceiving, many of which revolve around making better dietary choices.

However, sifting through the plethora of nutritional advice found in magazine articles, infertility blogs, internet stories, and well-meaning advice from friends and family can be overwhelming. All you want is to increase your chances of getting pregnant and having a healthy baby, but conflicting diet recommendations can leave you feeling exhausted and confused. Keto? Paleo? Mediterranean? Should you cut out sugar or caffeine? Go high-fat or low-fat? It's a dizzying array of do's and don'ts.

Regardless of the plethora of information available, it's essential to recognize that diet can indeed impact fertility. What you eat matters. Here are ten nutritional guidelines to enhance preconception fertility and improve the likelihood of a healthy pregnancy.

How Can I Improve My Chances of Conceiving?

1. Quit Smoking: This is the most significant step you can take to boost your chances of getting pregnant and ensuring a healthy pregnancy. Smoking can decrease sperm count, motility, and semen volume in men, while in women, moderate to heavy smoking can elevate follicle-stimulating hormone

(FSH) levels, potentially leading to ovulation issues and fertility problems.

2. Maintain a Healthy Weight: Both being over or underweight can hinder conception for both partners. Women who are underweight, overweight, or obese may experience ovulation dysfunction and an increased risk of miscarriage. In men, carrying excess weight can result in an accumulation of extra body tissue and heat around the testicles, which can have detrimental effects on both sperm production and motility.

3. Limit Alcohol Intake: Alcohol consumption during pregnancy can result in various birth defects. It's crucial to avoid alcohol when trying to conceive, as it can reduce the odds of pregnancy and increase the risk of miscarriage and fetal death. For men, alcohol consumption during conception attempts can impair sperm motility and semen volume.

4. Take Prenatal Vitamins: Women should take a prenatal DHA vitamin and 800 micrograms of folic acid daily to enhance fertilization and pregnancy chances. For men, a daily multivitamin and Coenzyme Q10 can help prevent oxidative stress in sperm, preserving DNA integrity and reducing sperm damage.

Optimizing Fertility through Nutrition
Enhancing fertility involves more than just tracking ovulation cycles; nutrition plays a pivotal role in fertility outcomes. Here's a breakdown of dietary strategies to boost fertility and increase the likelihood of conception.

Fertility-Boosting Foods
1. Whole Grains and High-Fiber Foods:
Go for whole grains over high-sugar carbs to

combat insulin resistance, which can disrupt ovulation. Whole grains, rich in fiber, help regulate blood sugar levels and support hormonal balance.

2. Clean Fruits and Vegetables: Choose organically grown produce or thoroughly wash conventionally grown fruits and vegetables to minimize pesticide exposure. Pesticides can interfere with hormone production, potentially impacting fertility.

3. Omega-3 Fatty Acids: Prioritize foods rich in omega-3 fatty acids, such as seafood, nuts, seeds (like chia and flax), and Brussels sprouts. Omega-3s improve egg quality, reduce inflammation, and support ovulation and a healthy pregnancy.

4. Plant-Based Protein: Replace red meat and poultry with plant-based protein sources like soy, beans, lentils, and quinoa. Plant-based proteins lower the risk of ovulatory disorders associated with excessive intake of omega-6 fatty acids found in animal-based proteins.

Plant-Based Diet for Fertility

Transitioning to a plant-based diet can enhance fertility by reducing intake of substances detrimental to reproductive health. Plant-based proteins offer numerous benefits, including a favorable fatty acid profile and lower risk of ovulatory disorders.

Foods to Limit or Avoid

1. Processed Foods: Limit consumption of processed meats, fast food, and microwave popcorn, which contain trans fats, animal fats, and additives linked to ovulatory infertility. Reheating foods in plastic containers increases exposure to endocrine-disrupting chemicals, potentially affecting embryo development.

2. Caffeine: Reduce or eliminate caffeine intake, as high consumption is associated with decreased fertility and increased risk of negative pregnancy outcomes. Excessive caffeine intake may lead to difficulties in conceiving and elevate the risk of miscarriage, fetal death, and stillbirth.

Seeking Assistance with Fertility

If you're facing challenges with conception or aiming to optimize nutrition and weight for fertility, consider consulting fertility experts that provides personalized guidance and cost-conscious treatment options to support couples on their journey to parenthood. From nutritional counseling to tailored treatment plans, they offer comprehensive support to enhance your chances of conceiving.

CHAPTER 4

BREAKFAST TO START YOUR DAY RIGHT

American Pancakes: When it comes to American pancakes, it's all about the bigger, the better! Just take a look at IHOP's colossal pancakes - they redefine the term huge.

American's love affair with pancakes goes beyond their sweet reputation. They're versatile, pairing perfectly with both sweet and savory toppings like bacon, eggs, and even fried chicken. And while they make a delicious breakfast, they can easily transition into a satisfying lunch. But amidst all the variations, nothing quite beats the simple pleasure of melted butter on top.

Ingredients:

• 200g self-rising flour

- 1 ½ tsp baking powder

- 1 tbsp golden caster sugar

- 3 large eggs

- 25 grams of melted butter, with additional butter for cooking

- 200ml milk

- Vegetable oil, for cooking

Method:

1. Combine self-raising flour, baking powder, golden caster sugar, and a pinch of salt in a large bowl.

2. Create a depression in the middle and incorporate eggs, melted butter, and milk. Blend thoroughly until achieving a smooth consistency.

3. Heat butter and oil in a frying pan, then pour rounds of batter. Cook until bubbles

start to appear, then flip the pancake and cook the opposite side.

4. Serve stacked with maple syrup and your favorite toppings.

Bacon and Eggs: Bacon and eggs are a quintessential American breakfast staple, often found alongside pancakes and waffles. They're incredibly versatile, featuring in various dishes like breakfast burritos or simply served with hash browns.

Ingredients:

• 8 eggs

• 1/2 cup cherry tomatoes

• Salt, to taste

• 150g bacon

• 1/4 cup parsley

• Black pepper, to taste

Method:

1. Fry bacon until crispy, then set aside.

2. In the same pan, cook eggs and cherry tomatoes.

3. Season eggs, garnish with parsley, and serve hot with bacon.

Scrambled Eggs: Scrambled eggs are a beloved breakfast choice worldwide, especially in America where they often accompany pancakes and bacon. They're incredibly versatile and can be customized with milk and cheese for added flavor.

Ingredients:

• 4 large eggs

• 1/4 cup milk

• Pinch of salt

- Pinch of pepper

- 2 tsp butter

Method:

1. Combine eggs, milk, salt, and pepper thoroughly by whisking them together.

2. Heat butter in a skillet, then pour in the egg mixture.

3. Gently pull and fold eggs until thickened and no liquid remains.

4. Serve immediately.

Eggs Benedict: Easily Elevate Your Morning with This Classic Dish

Have you ever wondered what exactly makes up the beloved breakfast or brunch staple known as Eggs Benedict? In essence, it's a delightful combination of poached eggs, toasted English muffins, and crispy bacon or Canadian bacon, all brought together with a luxurious hollandaise sauce. This ensemble of flavors and textures provides the perfect fuel to kick-start your day.

Ingredients:

• You have the option of using either 8 slices of bacon or 4 slices of Canadian bacon.

• 4 large eggs

• 2 teaspoons of white vinegar or alternatively rice vinegar

• 2 English muffins

• Butter

• Add two tablespoons of finely chopped parsley to use as a garnish.

For the hollandaise sauce:

• 10 tablespoons of unsalted butter (if using salted butter, skip the additional salt)

• 3 large egg yolks

- 1 tablespoon of lemon juice

- 1/2 teaspoon of kosher salt

- A small amount of cayenne pepper or Tabasco sauce

Method:

1. Cook the bacon:

- Warm a sizable skillet on medium-low temperature.

- Add the bacon slices and cook slowly, turning occasionally, until browned and crisp (about 10 minutes).

- Once cooked, remove the bacon from the pan and place it on a paper towel to absorb excess fat.

2. Prepare the poaching water

- While the bacon is cooking, bring a large saucepan filled two-thirds with water to a boil.

•Add vinegar to the water and bring it back to a boil, then reduce the heat to a gentle simmer.

3. Make the hollandaise sauce

• Gently melt the unsalted butter.

• In a blender, combine the egg yolks, lemon juice, salt, and blend until the mixture lightens in color.

• With the blender on low, slowly add the melted butter until the sauce is smooth and creamy.

• Adjust the seasoning with additional salt or lemon juice if needed, then transfer the sauce to a warm container.

4. Poach the eggs

• Gently crack each egg into an individual small bowl before delicately transferring them into the gently simmering water.

• Cook for approximately 4 minutes until the egg whites are firm but the yolks remain slightly liquid.

• Use a slotted spoon to carefully lift the poached eggs out of the water, allowing any excess water to drain away.

5. Toast the English muffins

• Toast the English muffins until they reach a golden brown color.

6. Assemble the Eggs Benedict

• Spread butter on one side of each English muffin.

• Top with bacon slices followed by a poached egg.

• Spoon hollandaise sauce over the eggs and sprinkle with chopped parsley.

• Serve immediately and enjoy this indulgent breakfast treat!

Avocado Toast: An Expedient and Nutritious Breakfast Choice

Avocado toast may not be everyone's cup of tea, but it certainly has its fans, thanks to its nutritious blend of carbs and healthy fats. Perfect for those busy mornings, this simple recipe can be whipped up in just five minutes.

Ingredients:

- ½ small avocado

- ½ teaspoon fresh lemon juice

- ⅛ teaspoon Kosher salt

- ⅛ teaspoon freshly ground black pepper

- 1 slice whole grain bread, toasted

- ½ teaspoon extra-virgin olive oil

- Optionally, sprinkle Maldon sea salt flakes or red pepper flakes on top for added flavor and garnish.

Directions:

1. In a small bowl, mash the avocado with lemon juice, salt, and pepper using the back of a fork.

2. Spread the mashed avocado mixture onto the toasted bread.

3. Drizzle with olive oil and sprinkle with desired toppings like sea salt flakes or red pepper flakes, if using.

4. Enjoy your quick and nutritious avocado toast!

Breakfast Burritos: Seeking a hearty morning meal? Look no further than breakfast burritos! Much like other American breakfast classics, burritos boast staples like bacon, ham, sausages, scrambled eggs, and more. You also have the option of including a single slice of cheese. The options are limitless, with your creativity being the only boundary.

Ingredients:

• 3 tablespoons vegetable oil

• Four cups, which is equivalent to 12 ounces, of frozen shredded hash brown potatoes, sourced from a 30-ounce bag.

• 8 eggs

• One container, measuring 4 ounces, of Old El Paso Chopped Green Chiles.

• 1/2 teaspoon salt

• 1/2 teaspoon pepper

• 6 fully cooked breakfast sausage links, cut into 1/4-inch pieces

• One packet, weighing 11 ounces, of Old El Paso Flour Tortillas specifically designed for making burritos, containing 8 tortillas.

• Two cups of shredded Mexican cheese blend, which typically amounts to around 8 ounces.

Directions:

1. In a 12-inch nonstick skillet, heat 2 tablespoons of oil over medium-high heat. Add frozen hash brown potatoes in an even layer and press down lightly. Allow the potatoes to cook undisturbed for 7 minutes. Afterward, drizzle them with the remaining tablespoon of oil, then flip them over. Continue cooking for an extra 6 to 8 minutes, or until they are golden brown on both sides and thoroughly heated. Transfer them to a medium bowl and cover with foil to retain warmth. Clean the skillet.

2. In a large bowl, beat eggs, green chiles, salt, and pepper until well blended. In the identical skillet over medium-high heat, cook the sausage for 2 to 3 minutes, stirring often, until

it is nicely browned. Stir in the egg mixture and cook for another 2 to 3 minutes, stirring occasionally, until scrambled.

3. To prepare the burritos, place a line of hash browns down the center of each tortilla. Add cheese and the scrambled egg mixture on top. Roll each tortilla tightly to enclose the filling securely. Serve promptly or freeze for later use.

Many of our favorite breakfast foods are carb-loaded, making it tricky for those on low carb or ketogenic diets. Luckily, there are plenty of flavorful, low carb breakfast options available. Here are some recipes to kick start your day the right way.

1. Spinach and Goat Cheese Omelet

Healthy beginnings: tempting low-carb breakfast recipes

Indulge in a creamy omelet filled with spinach and goat cheese for a satisfying breakfast.

Ingredients:

- 3 large eggs

- 2 tbsp (30 mL) heavy cream

- 1 cup (30g) spinach

- 1 oz (28g) goat cheese

- 1 tbsp (14g) butter

- Salt and pepper to taste

Directions:

- Beat together eggs, heavy cream, salt, and pepper until well combined.

- Sauté spinach in butter until wilted.

• Pour the egg mixture into the pan and proceed with cooking.

• Add spinach and goat cheese, then fold and serve.

2. Veggie Frittata

Enjoy a colorful frittata packed with veggies and feta cheese, baked to perfection.

Ingredients:

• 6 large eggs

• 1/3 cup (80 mL) milk

• 4 cloves garlic, minced

• 2 cups (60g) kale, chopped

• 2 cups (300g) bell peppers, chopped

• 1 oz (28g) crumbled feta

• 1 tbsp (15 mL) olive oil

Directions:

• Combine eggs, milk, minced garlic, and a pinch of salt and pepper, blending until smooth and well-mixed.

• Sauté kale and bell peppers in olive oil.

• Pour in egg mixture and sprinkle with feta.

• Bake until firm, then cut into slices and serve.

3. Baked Avocado Eggs

Elevate your breakfast with baked avocado filled with eggs and your favorite toppings.

Ingredients:

• 1 avocado

• 2 large eggs

• Salt and pepper to taste

• Optional toppings: bacon bits, cheese, chives, cilantro, tomatoes

Directions:

• Slice avocado and remove pit.

• Crack an egg into each half.

• Season, add toppings, and bake until desired doneness.

4. Shakshuka

Savor the rich flavors of this Middle Eastern dish featuring poached eggs in a spicy tomato sauce.

Ingredients:

• 6 large eggs

• 1 onion, diced

• 1 red bell pepper, diced

• 3 cloves garlic, minced

• 28 oz (794g) crushed tomatoes

- Salt, pepper, paprika, red chili powder, cumin to taste

- 2 oz (57g) crumbled feta

- Fresh cilantro, chopped

Directions:

• Sauté onions and bell peppers, then add tomatoes and spices.

• Create indentations in the sauce and gently place cracked eggs within each indentation.

• Cover the dish and allow the eggs to cook until they reach the desired level of doneness.

• Top with feta and cilantro before serving.

5. Broccoli and Bacon Crustless Quiche

Enjoy a hearty quiche packed with broccoli, bacon, and cheddar cheese.

Ingredients:

• 6 large eggs

• 1 cup (240 mL) milk

• 1 cup (90g) broccoli, chopped

• 4 slices bacon, chopped

• 3/4 cup (85g) shredded cheddar cheese

• 2 tbsp (30 mL) olive oil

• Salt and pepper to taste

Directions:

• Cook bacon until crispy, then sauté broccoli.

• Spread bacon and broccoli in a pie dish.

• Whisk eggs, milk, salt, and pepper, then pour over the veggies.

• Sprinkle cheese over the mixture and bake it until it reaches a firm, set consistency.

6. Zucchini Egg Nests

Revamp your breakfast routine with zucchini egg nests – a delightful low-carb option packed with flavor.

Ingredients:

• 2 zucchinis, spiralized

- 2 large eggs

- 1 tbsp (30 mL) olive oil

- Salt and pepper to taste

- Optional toppings: feta cheese, sliced avocado, red pepper flakes

Directions:

- Preheat oven to 350°F (180°C).

- Sauté spiralized zucchini in olive oil until tender.

- Arrange zucchini in nests in a skillet, crack an egg into each, sprinkle with salt and pepper, and bake for 5 minutes.

- Top with desired toppings and serve.

7. Veggie Egg Cups

Start your day right with these veggie-packed egg cups, a convenient and nutritious breakfast option.

Ingredients:

- 12 large eggs

- 1/3 cup (80 mL) milk

- 1/4 cup (29 grams) red onion, diced

- 1 cup (70 grams) mushrooms, diced

- Dice 1 cup (150 grams) of bell peppers.

- 1/2 cup (90 grams) tomatoes, diced

- 1 cup (110 grams) shredded cheese

- 2 tbsp (30 mL) olive oil

- Salt and pepper to taste

Directions:

- Preheat oven to 350°F (180°C).

- Cook vegetables in olive oil until they're tender.

- Distribute vegetables and cheese evenly into a greased muffin tin.

• In a bowl, mix eggs, milk, salt, and pepper, then pour into each muffin cup.

• Bake until firm, then let it cool down prior to serving.

8. Scrambled Eggs with Turkey Sausage

Enjoy a protein-packed breakfast with scrambled eggs and savory turkey sausage.

Ingredients:

• 2 large eggs

• 2 tbsp (30 mL) heavy cream

• 1 tbsp (14 grams) butter

• Salt and pepper to taste

• 1 turkey sausage patty

Directions:

• Combine eggs, heavy cream, salt, and pepper in a bowl and whisk them together until well blended.

• Melt butter in a pan over medium-low heat, add egg mixture, and scramble until mostly cooked.

• Cook turkey sausage patty in a separate pan over medium heat and serve alongside scrambled eggs.

CHAPTER 5

RAPID AND NUTRITIOUS LUNCH SUGGESTIONS FOR HECTIC SCHEDULES

In today's fast-paced world, making time for a nourishing midday meal can pose a challenge. This assortment of speedy and nutritious lunch options aims to alleviate the pressures of hectic schedules. Not only are these recipes delicious, but they're also tailored to suit individuals with jam-packed agendas, whether they're working remotely or constantly on the go.

Avocado and Chickpea Salad
Ingredients:

• 1 ripe avocado, diced

• Chickpeas, one can (15 ounces) - chickpeas from a single can, washed and thoroughly drained

• Cherry tomatoes, halved

• Cucumber, diced

• Finely chopped red onion

• Chopped fresh cilantro

• Season with your desired amount of olive oil, lemon juice, salt, and pepper.

Instructions: Combine diced avocado, chickpeas, cherry tomatoes, cucumber, red onion, and cilantro in a bowl. Drizzle with olive oil and lemon juice. Season with salt and pepper. Gently toss to mix.

Quinoa and Vegetable Stir-Fry
Ingredients:

• Cooked quinoa

• Diced assortment of vegetables (including bell peppers, broccoli, and carrots)

• Minced garlic

• Soy sauce

• Sesame oil

• Chopped green onions

• Sesame seeds for garnish

Instructions: Stir-fry mixed vegetables and garlic in a pan put cooked quinoa and flavor it with soy sauce and sesame oil according to your preference. Mix well. Sprinkle with chopped scallions and sesame seeds for a finishing touch.

**Mediterranean Wrap
Ingredients:**

• Whole wheat tortilla

• Hummus

- Grilled chicken strips

- Sliced cherry tomatoes

- Thinly sliced cucumber

- Chopped Kalamata olives

- Crumbled feta cheese

- Fresh spinach leaves

Instructions: Spread hummus on a whole wheat tortilla. Layer with grilled chicken strips, cherry tomatoes, cucumber, Kalamata olives, feta cheese, and spinach leaves. Roll tightly.

Fancy Tomato Sandwiches
Ingredients:

- 3/4 cup of softened salted butter (equivalent to 1 1/2 sticks)

- 1/4 cup plus 2 tablespoons of freshly minced chives

• Two elongated baguettes, approximately 12 ounces each

• 8 ounces of Gruyère, Comté, or sharp Cheddar cheese, cut into slices about 1/4 inch thick

• 8 small to medium firm-ripe heirloom tomatoes, totaling 3 pounds altogether, with cores removed and sliced to a thickness of 1/4 inch

• ¾ teaspoon kosher salt

• Freshly ground black pepper

• 3 cups baby arugula

•Include 2 cups of crunchy fried onions, like those from French's brand.

Directions:

1. Mix butter and chives until smooth.

2. Slice baguettes horizontally. Spread chive butter on both cut sides.

3. Layer cheese, tomatoes seasoned with salt and pepper, arugula, and onions on bottom baguette halves.

4. Place top baguette halves. Slice each sandwich crosswise into 8 pieces for appetizers or 4 pieces for a main course.

Crispy Chickpea Pita
Ingredients

• 3 tablespoons of olive oil

• 2 15.5-ounce cans of chickpeas, rinsed and drained

• 3 tablespoons of lemon juice squeezed from fresh lemons

• ¼ cup of roughly chopped fresh flat-leaf parsley, plus additional whole parsley leaves

• ¾ teaspoon of kosher salt

- ½ teaspoon of black pepper

- 4 plum tomatoes, diced

- 4 pitas or flatbread pieces, warmed

- 1 8-ounce container of hummus

- 1 small red onion, thinly sliced

- 1 teaspoon of hot sauce like Tabasco or a similar brand

- ½ cup of plain yogurt

- 1 lemon, cut into wedges

Directions

1. Warm 2 tablespoons of olive oil in a skillet on medium-high heat. Add chickpeas and cook, stirring occasionally, until lightly browned, approximately 5 minutes.

2. Remove from heat and toss with lemon juice, chopped parsley, ½ teaspoon of salt, and ¼ teaspoon of pepper.

3. In a small bowl, mix whole parsley leaves, tomatoes, and remaining olive oil, salt, and pepper.

4. Divide warmed bread among 4 plates and spread with hummus. Top with chickpea mixture, onion, and hot sauce. Serve with parsley salad, yogurt, and lemon wedges.

Chicken Tortilla Crunch Salad

Ingredients

• Canola oil for grill grates

• 1 pound of boneless, skinless chicken thighs (4 thighs)

• Add 2 tablespoons of either fajita or taco seasoning mix.

• 1 ¼ teaspoon of kosher salt, divided

• Use either 6 cups of shredded napa cabbage from one head of cabbage or a 14-ounce package of coleslaw mix.

- 1 red bell pepper, thinly sliced

- ¼ cup of mayonnaise

- ¼ cup of salsa

- 2tablespoons of sour cream

- Two cups of corn tortilla chips, crushed.

- 1cup of roughly chopped fresh cilantro, plus additional for serving

- 2 ounces of queso fresco or feta cheese, crumbled (about 1/2 cup)

- ¼ cup of roasted, salted pumpkin seeds (pepitas)

Directions

1. Coat the grill grates with oil and heat them up to a medium-high temperature, around 400°F to 450°F. Season the chicken thighs with fajita seasoning and a pinch of salt.

2. Cook the chicken on the oiled grates until it's thoroughly cooked, typically around 4 to 5 minutes per side. Then, transfer it to a plate and allow it to cool for about 15 minutes before serving.

3. Mix together cabbage and bell pepper in a large bowl. In a separate small bowl, blend mayonnaise, salsa, sour cream, and the remaining ¾ teaspoon of salt. Combine this mixture with the cabbage and bell pepper, tossing until they're evenly coated.

4. Slice the chicken thinly and add it to the cabbage mixture along with the tortilla chips. Toss everything together to combine. Transfer the mixture to a bowl or plates, then sprinkle with cheese and pepitas on top. Finish by garnishing with cilantro.

CHAPTER 6

EASY DINNER IDEAS FOR SIMPLE, SATISFYING EVENINGS

Chicken-Fried Steak with Creamy Gravy Ingredients

• 1teaspoon of garlic powder

• 4 and half teaspoons of kosher salt (plus more to taste)

• 2teaspoons of black pepper (plus more for garnish)

• 4cube steaks (6 ounces each)

• 2/3 cup of finely crushed buttery round crackers (like Ritz, from about 16 to 18 crackers)

• 1 and a half cups plus 3 tablespoons of all-purpose flour (divided)

- 2large eggs

- 2 and a half cups plus 2 tablespoons of whole milk (divided)

- 3cups of vegetable oil

Directions

1. **Season the steaks:** Preheat the oven to 200°F. Mix garlic powder, 3 teaspoons of salt, and 1 and a half teaspoons of pepper in a small bowl. Sprinkle 2 and a half teaspoons of the seasoning mix evenly over both sides of the steaks.

2. **Prepare breading stations:** Combine crushed crackers, 1 and a half cups of flour, and the remaining seasoning mix in a shallow bowl. Whisk eggs and 2 tablespoons of milk in another shallow bowl until well combined.

3. **Coat the steaks:** Heat oil in a large cast-iron skillet over medium to 325°F. Dredge

each steak in the flour mixture, then dip into the egg mixture, and coat again with flour mixture.

4. Fry the steaks: Carefully place 2 steaks in the hot oil and fry until golden brown on both sides, about 3 to 5 minutes per side. Transfer to a paper towel-lined plate, sprinkle with salt, then keep warm in the oven. Repeat with the remaining steaks.

5. Make the gravy: Drain fat from the skillet, reserving 1/4 cup drippings mixture. Return reserved drippings mixture and solids to the skillet over medium-low heat. Whisk in 3 tablespoons of flour and cook until bubbly, about 1 minute. Gradually whisk in the remaining 2 and a half cups of milk. Cook over low heat until the mixture becomes thicker, typically taking around 6 to 7 minutes. Stir in remaining salt and pepper.

6. Serve: Transfer steaks to a serving platter and serve immediately with warm gravy. Garnish with black pepper.

Mississippi Pork Chops

Tangy Pork Chops with Pepperoncini Peppers

Ingredients

- 4 bone-in rib-cut pork chops (10 ounces each, 1 to 1 and a quarter inches thick)
- 2 teaspoons of buttermilk ranch dressing mix (from a 1-ounce envelope)
- 1 teaspoon of kosher salt
- Half a teaspoon of black pepper
- 2 tablespoons of canola oil
- Quarter cup of unsalted butter
- One petite red onion, sliced thinly (equivalent to roughly 2 cups).

- 1 cup of jarred pepperoncini salad peppers, plus half a cup of liquid from the jar (divided)
- 2 teaspoons of jarred beef stock base (like Better Than Bouillon)
- 2 teaspoons of cornstarch
- Quarter cup of finely chopped mixed fresh herbs (such as parsley, dill, and chives)

Directions

1. Preheat the oven to 350°F. Season pork chops with ranch dressing mix, salt, and pepper. Warm oil in a sizable cast-iron skillet on high heat. Sear pork chops on each side until golden brown, approximately 8 minutes. Then, move them to a plate.

2. Reduce heat to medium-high. Melt butter in the skillet, then cook onion until slightly softened, about 4 minutes.

3. Whisk together pepperoncini liquid, beef stock base, and water. Return pork to skillet, add pepperoncini peppers and liquid mixture.

4. Bake until pork reaches 140°F, about 10 to 12 minutes. Transfer pork to a platter, keeping gravy in the skillet.

5. Simmer gravy over medium-high heat. Whisk cornstarch with water and add to the gravy. Cook until thickened, about 2 minutes. Stir in herbs. Spoon over pork chops and serve.

Bourbon Chicken: A Flavorful Delight
What Is Bourbon Chicken?

Bourbon chicken is a delightful sautéed dish featuring a sweet-savory sauce infused with ketchup, brown sugar, honey, soy sauce, apple cider vinegar, spices, and, of course, bourbon. Traditionally served over rice, this dish can also be enjoyed with a medley of sautéed vegetables.

Origins of Bourbon Chicken

The specific origins of this cuisine are somewhat uncertain. Many tales attribute its creation to Bourbon Street in New Orleans, which lends its name to the dish. Hence, Bourbon chicken is often associated with Cajun cuisine. However, alternative narratives suggest that it was crafted by a Chinese-American eatery situated on Bourbon Street, aiming to create a fusion dish tailored to local tastes. Regardless of its genesis, Bourbon chicken has become a beloved culinary gem across the United States, particularly in the Southern regions, cherished for its tantalizing flavor profile.

Ingredients for Bourbon Chicken

While the ingredient list may seem lengthy, most of these items are kitchen staples you likely already have on hand:

• **Boneless, skinless chicken thighs:** This cut ensures tender and succulent chicken pieces after sautéing.

• **Kosher salt and black pepper:** Essential for seasoning the chicken.

• **Cornstarch:** Used both for coating the chicken and thickening the sauce.

• **Canola oil:** Ideal for cooking the chicken.

• **Light brown sugar:** Adds a rich caramel sweetness to the sauce.

• **Apple juice:** Offers a touch of tartness and natural sweetness.

• **Unsalted chicken broth:** Contributes to the sauce's depth; opt for unsalted to control the dish's saltiness.

• **Bourbon:** Provides a distinctive flavor; can be substituted with apple juice if preferred.

• **Lower-sodium soy sauce:** Balances the flavors without overwhelming saltiness.

• **Honey:** Imparts subtle floral undertones, elevating the dish's complexity.

• **Ketchup:** Enhances umami notes with a hint of sweetness.

• **Apple cider vinegar:** Adds brightness and acidity to the sauce.

• **Onion powder and ground ginger:** Infuse depth and warmth into the flavor profile.

• **Tap water:** Used to create a slurry with cornstarch for thickening the sauce.

• **Thinly sliced scallions:** Sprinkled over the dish before serving, offering a fresh, green contrast.

• **Steamed white rice:** The perfect accompaniment to soak up the delectable sauce.

Directions for Preparation

1. In a medium bowl, toss chicken pieces with salt, pepper, and 2 tablespoons of cornstarch until evenly coated.

2. Warm a tablespoon of oil in a sizable nonstick skillet over medium to high heat. Cook half of the chicken pieces until browned on all sides, about 3 to 4 minutes per side. Move the cooked chicken to a plate and proceed with the remaining oil and chicken in the same manner.

3. Meanwhile, whisk together brown sugar, apple juice, chicken broth, bourbon, soy

sauce, honey, ketchup, vinegar, onion powder, and ground ginger in a medium bowl.

4. Pour the sauce mixture into the skillet and bring to a boil over medium-high heat for about 1 minute. Add the chicken back to the skillet, including any juices that have collected. Simmer the mixture, stirring occasionally, until it thickens by half and nicely coats the back of a spoon, which should take around 4 minutes.

5. In a small bowl, whisk together 1 1/2 teaspoons of water and the remaining 1 1/2 teaspoons of cornstarch. Stir this mixture into the sauce in the skillet and simmer until the sauce thickens and glazes the chicken, about 1 minute.

6. Sprinkle the dish evenly with sliced scallions and serve hot over steamed white rice. Enjoy the flavorful indulgence of Bourbon Chicken!

Pulled Pork Loaded Baked Potatoes
Ingredients:

• 8 medium russet potatoes (about 8 oz. each)

• 2 tablespoons olive oil

• 1 large yellow onion, thinly sliced

• One sizable red bell pepper, sliced thinly in a vertical manner.

• 1/4 teaspoon kosher salt

• 1/4 teaspoon black pepper

• About 2 cups of shredded Monterey Jack cheese, approximately 8 ounces.

• Roughly 1 and a half pounds of warmed pulled smoked pork.

• Coarsely crush around 2 cups of corn chips, like Fritos.

• 2 small ripe avocados, diced

- 1 1/2 cups barbecue sauce

- 1/4 cup chopped fresh cilantro

- 1 (14-oz.) package coleslaw mix

- 3/4 cup white barbecue sauce

Directions:

1. Begin by preheating the oven to 400°F. Then, arrange the potatoes on a generously-sized baking sheet lined with aluminum foil. Let them bake until they reach a delightful tenderness, typically around 45 minutes.

2. While the potatoes are baking, take a large skillet and set it over medium heat. Pour in a bit of olive oil and let it warm up. Once heated, toss in the onion slices and sauté them, stirring regularly, until they become soft and acquire a light brown hue, usually taking about 5 to 7 minutes. Following this, introduce the bell pepper into the skillet and continue to stir-cook for an additional 5 minutes. Once done, remove the skillet from the heat and season the mixture with salt and black pepper to taste.

3. Now, onto assembling the baked potatoes: Make a lengthwise incision down the center of each potato, ensuring not to slice all the way through. With gentle pressure, press the sides to create an opening. Tenderly mash the cooked potato flesh and nudge it towards the opening. Next, generously layer on the cheese, pork, onion-pepper mix, crushed corn chips, and diced avocado. For the finishing touch, drizzle some barbecue sauce over the top and sprinkle with cilantro.

4. Make coleslaw: Toss together coleslaw mix and white barbecue sauce. Serve with pork-stuffed potatoes.

Sheet Pan Greek Chicken with Roasted Potatoes
Ingredients:

• 2 teaspoons onion powder

• 2 teaspoons kosher salt

• 2 teaspoons dried thyme

• 1 teaspoon black pepper

- 1/4 teaspoon ground cinnamon

- 1/4 teaspoon ground nutmeg

- 1/4 cup of freshly chopped flat-leaf parsley, split into portions.

- Three teaspoons of freshly chopped oregano leaves, split into separate portions.

- 1/4 cup extra-virgin olive oil

- Four bone-in, skin-on chicken breasts, each weighing around 12 ounces, and trimmed.

- Eight slender lemon slices, sourced from two lemons.

- Use about 1 1/2 pounds of Yukon Gold potatoes, halved lengthwise (approximately 1 1/2 inch in diameter).

- Chop 1 tomato to yield about 1/2 cup of chopped tomato.

- Coarsely chop 1/2 cup of Kalamata olives.

• Crumble about 2 ounces of feta cheese, which should amount to roughly 1/4 cup when crumbled.

Directions:

Begin by preheating your oven to 400°F, ensuring the rack is positioned approximately 8 inches from the heat source. In a mini food processor, blend together onion powder, salt, thyme, pepper, cinnamon, nutmeg, 2 tablespoons of parsley, and 2 teaspoons of oregano until thoroughly combined. Next, add olive oil to the mixture and pulse until everything is well incorporated.

2. On a rimmed baking sheet, place the chicken and lemon slices. Evenly rub the chicken with 1/4 cup of the herb mixture. Then, toss the potatoes with the remaining herb mixture. Arrange the coated potatoes around the chicken and lemon slices on the baking sheet. Roast until a thermometer

inserted into the thickest part of the chicken reads 155°F and the potatoes are tender, typically around 30 minutes.

3. After roasting, increase the oven temperature to broil. Broil the chicken and potatoes until the skin of the chicken is browned and crispy, which usually takes about 5 minutes. Once done, remove the baking sheet from the oven and let it sit for 5 to 10 minutes. Finally, sprinkle the roasted chicken and potatoes with the chopped tomato, olives, crumbled feta cheese, and the remaining parsley and oregano.

Creamy Kale and Pasta Bake
Ingredients:

• 4 quarts water

• 1/4 cup plus 1 1/2 tsp. kosher salt, divided

• 1 (16-oz.) package chopped fresh kale

• 4 cups whole milk

• Cut 6 tablespoons of cold salted butter into pieces.

• Chop enough yellow onion to yield 1 cup (usually from 1 onion).

• Measure out 6 tablespoons of all-purpose flour.

• Use a pre-shredded package of Monterey Jack cheese, typically 8 ounces (about 2 cups).

• Add 1 teaspoon of hot sauce, like Tabasco.

• Include 1/2 teaspoon of black pepper.

• Cook 8 ounces of medium-size shell pasta according to the directions on the package.

• 1/2 cup panko (Japanese-style breadcrumbs)

• 1 tablespoon olive oil

Directions:

1. To start, preheat the broiler, ensuring the oven rack is positioned 8 to 9 inches from the heat source. In a Dutch oven, bring 4 quarts of water and 1/4 cup of salt to a boil over high heat. Add the chopped kale and cook until tender, typically around 5 to 7 minutes. Once cooked, drain the kale and gently pat it dry with paper towels. Allow it to really cool for roughly 10 minutes or more.

2. While the kale is cooling, pour milk into a 1-quart glass measuring cup. Cover it with plastic wrap and microwave it on HIGH for 3 minutes.

3. In the same Dutch oven used for the kale, melt butter over medium heat. Add the chopped onion and cook, stirring occasionally, until tender, which usually takes

about 6 minutes. Afterward, incorporate the flour and continue whisking constantly for a duration of 2 minutes. Gradually whisk in the hot milk. Increase the heat to medium-high and allow the mixture to gently boil, whisking regularly. Continue to cook and whisk until the mixture thickens, approximately 6 minutes. Remove the Dutch oven from the heat and whisk in the cheese, hot sauce, pepper, and the remaining 1 1/2 teaspoons of salt. Roughly chop the cooled kale and fold it together with the cooked pasta into the cheese sauce. Transfer the mixture into a greased 11- x 7-inch baking dish.

4. Finally, combine the panko breadcrumbs with 1 tablespoon of olive oil and sprinkle this mixture evenly over the pasta. Broil until the breadcrumbs turn golden brown, typically 1 to 2 minutes. Serve the dish immediately.

CHAPTER 7

EXPLORING VEGETARIAN AND VEGAN DIET

Vegetarianism encompasses a range of dietary choices, from those abstaining from meat but consuming eggs and dairy (lacto-ovo vegetarians) to those avoiding all animal products, including honey (vegans). Raw foodists are individuals who adhere to a vegan diet primarily consisting of raw fruits, vegetables, legumes, sprouts, and nuts. Additionally, there are pescatarians who eat fish, lacto-vegetarians who consume dairy but not eggs, fruitarians who focus on fruits, nuts, seeds, and other plant foods, and macrobiotic followers who primarily eat grains but may include fish.

Flexitarians, on the other hand, are vegetarians who occasionally incorporate meat and fish into their diets.

Reasons for Embracing Vegetarianism

Many advocates of vegetarianism, such as Paul McCartney and Alec Baldwin, advocate for its health benefits and ethical considerations. They highlight concerns about the environmental impact and cruelty associated with animal agriculture.

While some Americans adopt vegetarian diets, the majority still consume meat or fish, as indicated by a 2018 Gallup poll where only five percent identified as vegetarians.

Vegetarianism and Health

Numerous medical professionals and nutritionists endorse diets rich in fruits, vegetables, whole grains, and nuts for their potential health advantages. Research suggests that reducing or eliminating red meat may lower the risk of heart disease. Furthermore, studies indicate that vegans or vegetarians may have a reduced risk of type 2 diabetes, along with lower levels of triglycerides, glucose, blood pressure, and body mass index (BMI).

Cancer Risk and Vegetarianism

Determining the impact of vegetarianism on cancer risk is complex due to the diversity within the vegetarian community. However, diets abundant in fiber, vitamins, minerals, is oflavones, and carotenoids appear to offer protection against diseases like cancer when part of a health-conscious lifestyle. For instance, an 11-year study in Germany observed lower mortality rates from stomach, colon, and lung cancers among vegetarians, particularly those adhering to the diet for over 20 years. Nevertheless, factors such as body weight and exercise likely influence these outcomes.

Nutritional Considerations for Vegetarians

While a meatless diet can be nutritious, vegetarians, especially vegans, must ensure adequate intake of vitamin B12, calcium, iron, and zinc.

The Academy of Nutrition and Dietetics underscores the concern regarding vitamin B12 deficiencies among vegetarians and vegans, given that this vitamin is exclusively present in animal-derived products. A lack of vitamin B12 can lead to anemia, blindness, muscle weakness, tingling, and numbness. To address this risk, vegans should include B12 supplements, fortified cereals, or veggie burgers in their diets. While some mushrooms contain B12, particularly in the outer peel, it's too early to consider them a reliable source of the vitamin.

Vegans and ovo-vegetarians (those who eat eggs but not dairy) should strive to get calcium from dark green vegetables, tofu, edamame, soy nuts, butternut squash, and calcium-fortified non-dairy alternatives to offset the deficiency in calcium intake. beverages or supplements to make up for the absence of calcium in their diets. Absorbable calcium is crucial for protecting against osteoporosis, or thinning bones.

Pregnant and lactating women who are vegan face more urgent nutrition warnings. Vitamin B12 deficiency, in particular, has been linked to impaired neurological development in infants nursed by vegetarian mothers. Deficiencies in vitamin D and calcium can also lead to bone demineralization in breastfeeding women.

Children under 5 reared on vegetarian and vegan diets can experience impaired growth due to potential vitamin B12 deficiency, leading to anemia, and vitamin D deficiency, which can cause rickets. DHA, an omega-3 fatty acid primarily found in fish, is crucial for optimal brain development in the first two years of life. Consulting a registered dietitian for a well-planned diet can help meet all nutritional needs.

Key Nutrients for Vegetarians and Vegans
The U.S. Department of Agriculture and the Academy of Nutrition and Dietetics offer dietary guidelines for vegetarians on their websites. Irrespective of the specific type of meat-free diet adhered to, vegetarians need to ensure they consume sufficient amounts of protein, iron, calcium, zinc, vitamin B12, riboflavin, alpha-linolenic acid, and vitamin D.

Below are several methods to integrate these essential nutrients into a vegetarian eating plan:

• Sources of protein in a vegetarian diet include tofu, edamame, tempeh, veggie burgers containing 5 grams of protein or more, beans, nuts, nut butters, eggs, and high-protein whole grains like quinoa, amaranth, and kamut.

• In a vegetarian diet, sources of iron may comprise eggs, fortified breakfast cereals, soy-based products, dried prunes, dried apricots, nuts, beans, legumes, and fortified whole wheat bread.

• Calcium: Cheese, yogurt, milk, edamame, tofu, almonds, sesame tahini, calcium-fortified orange juice, calcium-fortified non-dairy beverages like soy or almond milk, and dark green leafy vegetables like collard greens, spinach, and bok choy.

• Zinc sources in vegetarian diets encompass soybeans, soy milk, veggie meats, eggs, cheese, yogurt, fortified breakfast cereals, nuts, seeds, mushrooms, lentils, black-eyed peas, split peas, and wheat germ.

• Vitamin B12 can be obtained from soy-based beverages, select breakfast cereals, and fortified veggie meats.

• Riboflavin-rich foods include almonds, fortified cereals, cow's milk, yogurt, mushrooms, and soy milk.

• To boost your intake of Alpha-Linolenic Acid (a type of Omega-3), integrate canola oil, ground flaxseeds, flaxseed oil, walnuts, walnut oil, soybeans, and tofu into your eating habits.

Plant-based appetizers

Cake infused with the rich flavors of caramelized onion, crunchy walnut, and earthy spinach.

Ingredients:

Onion Marmalade:

• 2 tablespoons olive oil

• 4 large sweet onions (such as Vidalia or Walla Walla), thinly sliced (about 7 cups)

• 3 tablespoons balsamic vinegar

• 1 1/2 tablespoons light brown sugar

• 1 teaspoon finely chopped fresh thyme

Cake:

• 1 1/2 cups all-purpose flour

• 1 tablespoon baking powder

• 1 teaspoon kosher salt

• 1 teaspoon Aleppo pepper (or 1 teaspoon paprika and a pinch of cayenne pepper)

• 2 large eggs

• 1/2 cup low-fat Greek yogurt

- 5 tablespoons olive oil

- 1 cup coarsely chopped spinach

- 1/3 cup chopped toasted walnuts

Preparation:

1. For the Onion Marmalade: Heat olive oil in a Dutch oven over medium-high heat. Cook the onions over medium heat for approximately half an hour, stirring occasionally. Stir in balsamic vinegar, brown sugar, and thyme, then reduce heat to medium-low. Cook for about 40 minutes, or until onions are caramelized. Let cool.

2. For the Cake: Preheat oven to 350°F. Line a loaf pan with parchment paper, leaving ends hanging over the edges. Spray parchment with cooking spray.

3. In a bowl, whisk together flour, baking powder, salt, and Aleppo pepper. In another

bowl, whisk together eggs, yogurt, and olive oil. Stir egg mixture into flour mixture. Gently incorporate spinach, along with 1/2 cup of the Onion Marmalade and walnuts. Transfer the mixture into the prepared loaf pan and use a spatula to even out the top. Bake for 45 minutes, or until a knife inserted into the loaf comes out clean. Lift loaf from pan using the parchment paper and cool on a wire rack. If desired, accompany with any leftover Onion Marmalade for added flavor.

Oven-Baked Eggplant Fries
Ingredients:

- 1 large eggplant

- 2 eggs

- 1/2 cup oat flour

- 1/4 teaspoon sea salt

- 1/4 teaspoon pepper

- 1/4 cup nonfat Greek yogurt

- 2 tablespoons low-fat cottage cheese

- 1 teaspoon chipotle chili powder

- 1 packet Stevia

Preparation:

1. Heat your oven to 425°F and prepare a baking sheet by lining it with parchment paper.

2. In a bowl, whisk together the eggs with salt and pepper. In another bowl, put the flour.

3. Cut the eggplant into thick fries. Dip each piece into the egg mixture, then coat evenly with flour.

4.Lay out the eggplant fries on the baking sheet and bake for 25 minutes, remembering to flip them over halfway through the cooking time.

5.While the eggplant fries are baking, use a food processor to blend together yogurt, cottage cheese, chili powder, and Stevia until you achieve a smooth consistency.

6. Serve fries with dipping sauce.

BBQ Mushroom Sliders
Ingredients:

Pimento Cheese:

• 2 cups grated sharp cheddar cheese

• 2 ounces reduced-fat cream cheese

• 4 ounces jarred pimento peppers, drained

• 1 teaspoon hot sauce

• 1/2 teaspoon garlic powder

• 1/2 teaspoon vegan Worcestershire sauce

• 1/4 teaspoon ground black pepper

• 3 tablespoons reduced-fat mayonnaise

BBQ Mushrooms:

• 2 tablespoons vegetable oil

• One medium onion, finely chopped, yielding approximately one and a half cups.

• Six large portobello mushroom caps, with their stems and gills removed, should be halved and thinly sliced.

• 1/2 cup prepared barbecue sauce

Sliders:

• 16 slider rolls

• Include 32 slices of bread and butter pickles, and you can add extra for garnish if desired.

Preparation:

1. For preparing the Pimento Cheese: Combine all the listed ingredients in a small bowl, mashing them together with a fork. Once mixed, set the mixture aside.

2. To prepare the BBQ Mushrooms: Heat oil in a large skillet over medium-high heat. Add the finely diced onion to the skillet and sauté for approximately 2 minutes. Then, add the mushrooms and cook for approximately 8 minutes until they are tender. After cooking, remove the skillet from the heat, stir in the barbecue sauce, and set it aside.

3. For assembling the Sliders: On each roll's bottom, spread 1 tablespoon of the prepared Pimento Cheese and 1 tablespoon of the BBQ Mushrooms. Top with two slices of pickle and cover with the top half of the bun to complete the sliders.

Charred Tomato, Pepper, and Onion Crostini

Ingredients:

• 3 small tomatoes, halved and seeded (about 2 cups)

• 1 small onion, quartered

• One medium or two small bell peppers, cut in half lengthwise and seeds removed.

• 6 cloves garlic, peeled

• 2 tablespoons olive oil, plus extra for brushing bread slices

• 6 large slices ciabatta bread

• 6 tablespoons shredded basil leaves for garnish

Preparation:

1. Adjust the oven racks to the middle and lower positions. Preheat the oven broiler to high. Place parchment paper on top of two baking sheets, ensuring a thorough and complete coverage.

2. Place the tomatoes, onion, bell peppers, and garlic cloves on one of the prepared baking sheets. Drizzle them with 2

tablespoons of olive oil and toss to ensure they are evenly coated. Arrange the vegetables cut-side down, ensuring the garlic cloves are tucked under the tomatoes to prevent them from burning. Position the baking sheet on the middle oven rack and broil for 8 to 10 minutes, or until the tomato skins become charred, stirring the vegetables once during the process. After broiling, pulse the vegetables in a food processor until they are coarsely chopped.

3. Arrange the bread slices on the second parchment-lined baking sheet. Place them under the broiler on the lower rack for 2 minutes, or until they turn lightly golden. Flip the bread slices and broil for an additional 2 minutes.

4. Brush the bread slices with olive oil. Spread each slice with 1/4 cup of the tomato mixture

and sprinkle 1 tablespoon of basil over the top.

CHAPTER 8

BEST MOCKTAIL RECIPES FOR PREGNANCY

Grapefruit Lime Mockgarita
Ingredients:

• Ice

• 1/3 cup freshly squeezed grapefruit juice

• The liquid obtained from squeezing half of a lime freshly.

• 1/4 cup chilled filtered water

• 1 teaspoon of pure maple syrup

Instructions:

1. In a cocktail shaker, mix a handful of ice with grapefruit juice, lime juice, filtered water, and maple syrup.

2. Shake thoroughly.

3. Add 5-6 ice cubes to a serving glass, pour in the mocktail, and garnish with a lime slice.

Health benefits:

This mocktail provides a dual boost of vitamin C from the citrus juices, aiding immunity and collagen production for resilient skin. Additionally, the manganese from maple syrup supports fetal bone and cartilage development. Its hydrating properties are especially beneficial during pregnancy, as increased blood volume necessitates higher fluid intake.

Blueberry Chia Crush

Ingredients:

• 1/2 cup frozen blueberries

• 1/4 cup chilled filtered water

• The juice extracted from half of a lime freshly squeezed.

- 1/2 tablespoon chia seeds

- 1 teaspoon pure maple syrup

- 1/2 cup sparkling water

Instructions:

1. In a mini blender, blend blueberries, filtered water, lime juice, chia seeds, and maple syrup until smooth.

2. Transfer to a cocktail glass and let sit for 5 minutes.

3. Add 5-6 ice cubes and sparkling water.

4. Stir well and garnish with whole blueberries.

Health benefits:

Chia seeds provide iron and calcium crucial for pregnant women's blood volume expansion and fetal bone development, respectively. Their fiber aids in blood sugar regulation, prevents constipation, and alleviates hemorrhoids. Blueberries, rich in antioxidants, help manage blood pressure and prevent urinary tract infections.

Mango Mint Quencher
Ingredients:

• 3/4 cup fresh mango

• 1/2 tablespoon freshly squeezed lemon juice

• 1/2 cup pure coconut water

• 2-3 fresh mint leaves

• 4-5 ice cubes

Instructions:

1. Combine mango, lemon juice, coconut water, fresh mint leaves, and ice cubes in a blender. Blend until smooth.

2. Pour into a glass and garnish with fresh mint.

Health benefits:

Mangoes offer vitamins A and C, vital for immunity, while coconut water's potassium regulates blood pressure and reduces fluid retention and leg cramps. Mint can alleviate morning sickness symptoms.

Pina Mocklada
Ingredients:

- 3/4 cup frozen pineapple chunks

- 1/2 cup frozen banana slices

- 3/4 cup unsweetened coconut milk

- 1/4 teaspoon freshly grated ginger root

- 1 teaspoon blackstrap molasses

- 1/2 teaspoon unsweetened shredded coconut

Instructions:

1. Using a mini blender, combine pineapple, banana, coconut milk, ginger root, and blackstrap molasses. Keep blending up until the mixture is smooth and combined well .

2. Pour into a glass and garnish with unsweetened shredded coconut.

Health benefits:

Pineapple provides magnesium, combating fatigue and promoting relaxation and sleep, essential during pregnancy. Bananas contain vitamin B6, aiding in alleviating nausea and supporting fetal brain and nervous system development. Blackstrap molasses offers iron, fighting pregnancy fatigue and promoting healthy hormone production.

Pomegranate Cosmo
Ingredients:

• Ice

- 1/2 cup 100 percent pomegranate juice

- 1/4 cup chilled filtered water

- Juice from half a lemon

- 1 teaspoon pure maple syrup

- 1/4 teaspoon freshly grated ginger root

- Pomegranate seeds (for garnish)

Instructions:

1. Mix together ice, pomegranate juice, cold filtered water, lemon juice, maple syrup, and grated ginger root in a cocktail shaker.

2. Shake well.

3. Pour into a glass and garnish with a few whole pomegranate arils.

Health benefits:

Pomegranate juice consumption during pregnancy may safeguard the placenta from injury risks, as per research in the American

Journal of Physiology: Endocrinology and Metabolism. Pomegranate also provides vitamin K, crucial for proper blood clotting to prevent excessive bleeding. Additionally, freshly grated ginger root, rich in anti-inflammatory antioxidants, may help alleviate morning sickness.

CONCLUSION

In this concluding section, we take a moment to contemplate the path we've embarked on towards enhanced health and well-being. Across the pages of this book, we've delved into a variety of delectable and healthful recipes crafted specifically to cater to the distinct requirements of women. From hearty breakfasts to satisfying dinners and everything in between, these culinary creations have not only fueled our bodies but also uplifted our spirits.

However, this cookbook exceeds, mere recipe compilations; it serves as a manual for embracing a more health-conscious lifestyle. We've engaged in discussions regarding the significance of maintaining a balanced diet, and integrating self-care routines that foster holistic wellness. Additionally, we've tackled prevalent health issues that often affect women, providing insights and tactics for addressing them through dietary adjustments and lifestyle modifications.

As we draw the final curtain on this chapter, let's bear in mind that health encompasses not only our dietary choices but also our way of life. It involves discovering joy in cooking and sharing meals with our loved ones and cultivating mindfulness towards our bodies, treating them with the reverence and attention they deserve.

I trust that the Healthy Female Cookbook has served as a source of inspiration for instigating positive transformations in your life and has emboldened you to seize control of your well-being. May these recipes continue to nurture you as you traverse towards a healthier, more contented self.

www.ingramcontent.com/pod-product-compliance
Lightning Source LLC
Chambersburg PA
CBHW070811260726
48660CB00005B/1812